The Metabolic Detox: The Detox Diet Plan For Cleansing Your Body, Improving Your Health, And Achieving Your Health Goals

Table of Contents

Introduction

Detoxification is the natural process occurring in our body which helps in removing the toxic substances from our body and thus maintaining an optimal health. Detoxification involves elimination of various poisonous or non-useful substances from the body. A person's health mainly depends on the ability of the body to eliminate waste effectively. Though the healthy cells in our body try to detoxify themselves every day, it will be difficult to remove all the toxins when there is too much of the toxins present in the body. Our environment contains various pollutants and these pollutants reach our body through the air, water and food. Exposure of the human body to these pollutants for a long time can cause health problems. When there is excess amount of pollutants or toxins in our body, it gets accumulated in various tissues. A detox diet plan helps to cleanse the body system and provides the necessary support for cleansing the organ such as liver, digestive system and kidney. Toxic substances which are water soluble are easily eliminated from the body, however the fat soluble toxins requires the support of enzymes present in liver to neutralize them and to break them down

The Effect Of Toxins On Our Body

The accumulation of toxins in our body can affect the various systems in the body. The important signs of buildup of toxins in our body include: fatigueness, muscle weakness, acne, rashes, memory loss, fertility issues, and poor immune function. It has been also found that exposure to toxins in smaller quantities, but for a longer period of time can result in Parkinson's disease, leukemia, fibromyalgia and certain lymphomas. The metabolic detoxification involves a chain of enzymatic reactions that neutralizes the toxins and makes them soluble in water. These toxins are then transported to various secretory organs in the body and finally get eliminated from the body. The overload of toxins and lack of essential nutrients required for the detoxification activities of the body prevent the harmful compounds present in our body to undergo the transformation. Over time these harmful compounds will have an adverse effect on your body. In our body, the lymph and circulatory system helps in the detoxification of individual cells. The principle organ responsible for detoxification of the body is the liver. Intestine and kidneys assist the liver in this process. The toxins are excreted through the skin, lungs, kidneys, bowel etc. When the natural detoxification is overwhelmed by the toxins, your body will need detoxification through diet. When the toxins challenge over body symptoms like headache, constipation, acne, joint pain, stomach pain, are all expressed.

Who Can Get Benefited By Detoxification?

Detoxification energizes the body and improves the healing power of the body. Detoxification is particularly beneficial to people suffering from chronic conditions like allergies, anxiety, arthritis, chronic infections, diabetes, heart disease, digestive disorder, high blood pressure, depression, high cholesterol and obesity. Detoxification diet plans also help to reduce the health problems caused by environmental factors like cancer. Detoxification is an effective preventive measure to increase the general health, vitality and immunity to various diseases. If you already have any health issues it is necessary that you consult your doctor before starting on a detox diet. To get lasting results on detoxification, you need to continue a diet which is healthy, that is based on vegetables, fruits, lean protein and whole grains.

The Health Benefits Of Detoxification

Though detoxification can be done using various methods, using a diet plan is highly beneficial. Through this method you will be able to detoxify the body in a natural way and this method is not expensive. The benefits of detoxification achieved by different organs of the body are given below.

Benefits To Liver

- The liver is the major detoxifying organ in the body. Every day, liver is filtering the various chemicals and hormones from the blood stream and eliminates the wastes. Detoxification helps to remove all the toxins from the liver.

- The detoxification diet contains all the macro and micro nutrients needed for the proper functioning of the enzymatic pathways occurring in the liver. This will help to enhance the functioning of the liver.

- Detox diet repairs the damages to the liver cells and reduces inflammation of the liver and viral infections of the liver.

- Certain foods like carrots, beets, turmeric, artichokes cleanse and heal the liver cells.

- Most of the detox diet plans will avoid allergy causing food items such as dairy products, soy, gluten containing grains, etc. Eliminating the allergy causing foods reduces the inflammation of the intestinal lining. When we are regularly taking these food items, the intestinal walls are inflamed, leading to poor assimilation of nutrients from food.

- During detoxification diet, there are chances that the probiotic bacteria or the friendly intestinal bacteria get reintroduced into your system. These probiotic bacteria are essential for the proper digestion of food and to prevent the various infections caused by intestinal parasites. These bacteria help to prevent constipation. It also helps in proper bowel movement and elimination of wastes from the body.

- Detoxification reduces health issues like indigestion, diarrhea, bloating, and constipation. The detoxification diet provides rest to the intestine and improves the digestion and assimilation of food after detoxification.

- Detoxification using diet is extremely useful for people suffering from intestinal inflammation due to irritable bowel syndrome and Crohn's disease.

Benefits To Hormone Metabolism

- Various endocrine organs produce the hormones which control the activities of the cells. These hormones reach the liver after completing their function. Liver de- activates these hormones and prepares it for elimination. When the function of the liver and intestine improves by detoxification the metabolism of hormones is done more effectively by the body.

- Better hormone metabolism reduces the premenstrual syndrome, such as mood swings, tenderness of the breasts and menstrual cramps.

- Detoxification reduces accumulation of hormone and hormonal wastes in the body, thus it reduces menopausal symptoms such as irritability, hot flashes, fatigue, insomnia, mood swings etc.

- The improved hormone metabolism provides better energy level and better sex drive in people.

- Detoxification of the body improves the functioning of various endocrine glands. Detoxification improves the functioning of adrenal glands and thyroid glands. This will provide better stress management ability, better moods and improves hair growth.

Benefits To The Musculoskeletal System

- Your muscles and joints get benefited by regular detoxification of the body using the proper diet plan. The toxins get deposited in the fat tissues in the body first and then they show an affinity for joints and muscles.

- Detoxification improves blood circulation to the joints and helps in the removal of toxic chemicals present in the joints and provides nutrients from the detoxification diet. This will improve the strength of the muscles and joints.

- The detoxification diets are mostly anti-inflammatory and will contain good amounts of omega 3 fatty acids in it. This will reduce the inflammations of the joints and muscles. This will lead to more flexibility of the joints and less pain.

Benefits To Cardiovascular System

- Detoxification reduces the lipid and cholesterol level in the body. The detox diet mainly consists of high fiber, low fat and low sugar food items which reduces the cholesterol and lipid level.

- The reduced level of cholesterol and lipids decreases the risk of cardiovascular problems.

- Detoxification helps to clear the blood vessels and improves the blood circulation

The Seven Day Detox Diet Plan

The seven day detox plan is the perfect diet plan that you can think of to detoxify the important organs of your body like liver, kidneys and bowel and at the same time improve your health and also achieve health goals set by you. It is the perfect way to lose weight without missing out on the nutrients that your body needs every day. If you are looking to fast track your health and to get your body free from toxins and unnecessary waste, then a complete seven day cleanse of your body is highly recommended. All you need to do is to follow this safe and very effective seven day detox diet plan and you will look in better shape at the end of the program.

Preparation for the Seven Day Diet Plan

The first and foremost thing that you need to do is to get yourself prepared for the seven day diet plan. You should choose a week that is devoid of any wedding anniversaries or birthday parties or get together and other occasions as this might ruin your seven day detox diet plan. You should be free from all kinds of foods and drinks for the entire seven days. You might also experience a cleansing reaction in the first couple of days of your detox plan as your body is getting adjusted to the new diet plan. You might experience sudden headaches, body tiredness as well as loose bowel movements. This is just because of the withdrawal of certain food items from your daily menu and there is nothing to get worried about. Make it a habit to drink at least 2.5 to 3 liters of water every day before your detox diet week as it will help in stimulating your detoxifying organs and keep them ready for the detox week ahead. The following diet is not a strict and a stubborn diet plan and gives you a wide variety of options to try out during your seven day detox diet program.

Foods to Include in the Plan

The following are the foods that you need to include in your plan:

- **Fruits**

It would be better for you to take any fresh fruit or all fresh fruits that you like during the seven day detox diet plan. Try to stick to just fresh fruits. But, you can also consume frozen or dried or canned fruits. Some of the common fruits that you need to include in your diet plan are:

  o Apples

  o Bananas

- Oranges

- Pears

- Raisins

- Sultanas

- Mango

- Pineapple

- Strawberries

- Raspberries

- Melons

- Peaches

- Blackcurrants

- Kiwi fruit

- Grapefruit

- **Vegetables**

You need to include a lot of vegetables in your seven day detox diet plan to help you cleanse your important body organs. You can go for canned or frozen vegetables. But, it would be ideal for you to stick to the fresh vegetable diet. Some of the vegetables that you should include in your diet are:

- o Carrots
- o Onions
- o Turnips
- o Sprouts
- o Beans
- o Mushrooms
- o Sweet corn
- o Cauliflower
- o Broccoli
- o Cabbage
- o Bell Peppers
- o Cucumber
- o Tomatoes
- o Spring Onions
- o Leeks

- Courgettes

- Lettuce

- **Other Foods That You Can Try Out**

If you are looking for a flexible seven day diet detox plan, then you can also try out some of the following foods as your mid day snacks or even for your lunch and dinner.

- Fresh fish like salmon, mackerel, cod, tuna, trout, swordfish, Dover sole, red mullet, halibut and so on.

- Nuts like pistachio, almonds, cashews, peanuts, pecans, hazelnuts, walnuts and pine nuts. Make sure that they are unsalted and that you just consume a handful of any nut as a mid day snack every day.

- Oats porridge or oats in slim milk or oats sweetened with honey and fruits

- Natural, fat free yoghurt

- Natural virgin olive oil and balsamic vinegar for salad dressing

- Brown rice and brown noodles, only twice or thrice for lunch or dinner for the entire week

- Herbal teas

- At least 2 to 2.5 liters of water every day

- **Foods To Avoid Completely**

The following are the foods that you should completely avoid during your detox plan. If you consume just a little bit of the following foods, then you are not going to get the health benefit that you are looking for. So, avoid all these foods during the one week detox plan.

- Milk, cream, cheese and eggs

- Butter, margarine and mayonnaise

- Red meat, chicken, beef, turkey and also processed meat foods

- Foods like biscuits, cakes, breads, pastries, croissants and so on that is made from white flour.

- Salted nuts, crispy and tasty snacks and savories

- Ice creams, chocolates, sauces, sweets, jam and sugar

- Alcohol, coffee and tea

- Pickles and sauces

- Aerated and fizzy drinks

The following is the seven day detox diet plan that you need to follow to achieve your health goals and to lose weight naturally. It is always better to start the day with fresh lemon juice as it is the ideal one that will kick start the digestion and also help in early cleansing of the body. Make sure that you start every day with a glass of fresh lemon juice without salt and sugar. You can add a dash of organic honey to the lemon juice. You can also occasionally squeeze a fresh lemon juice into a cup of hot boiling herbal or green tea and consume it early in the morning. Make sure that you also exercise for an hour every day during your detox plan. It will help in increasing the lymph flow and blood circulation in your body as well as remove all the toxins in your body through sweat. You can jog, walk uphill, swim, do yoga or even attend a spin class.

Day 1

The first day of your seven day detox diet plan should only be about fluids. You are sure to feel a little bit dizzy or fade away due to its liquid diet. All you need to do is to drink plenty of water to keep you hydrated. Some of the liquid diets that you can have during the day are:

- o Prepare fresh fruit and vegetable juices by either mixing two or three fresh fruits or fresh vegetables together in a blender. You can also think of going for a single fruit juice or a single vegetable juice.

- o You can also think of a combination of detox juices like carrots and apples or raspberries and peaches or any other fruit and fruit or fruit and vegetable combination that you would like to try out.

- o You can also take two to three cups of hot unsweetened green tea and add a pinch of ginger juice or lemon juice or dandelion or fennel to help in better detoxification of your body.

- o You can also think of taking vegetable broth during your first day detox plan. All you need is to cut some of the fresh organic vegetables into dices and boil them in clean and pure water and simmer for about 15 to 20 minutes. Do not add salt to this broth. Discard the vegetables and drink the broth two to three times throughout the day.

Day 2

Day two is also similar to day one, which is drinking plenty of fluids, as much as you want. The only change in the menu is that you can eat a portion of any of the fruits that you like when you feel hungry. As fruits are alkaline in nature, they will help in neutralizing the acidic waster that the body produces due to detoxification. Fruits are also a rich source of fiber and hence will help in removing some of the decayed material from your intestines and you will feel lighter after your diet program. Some of the foods that you can eat in raw state are:

- o Apples are a rich source of pectin that will help in easily removing toxins from your body and it also contains tartaric acid that will help in proper digestion.

- o Pineapples and mangoes are said to contain the bromelain enzyme that helps in producing the acids that will destroy the bad bacteria in the gut and will also encourage the growth of good bacteria in your body. It will also help in proper digestion and repairing of the worn out tissues. Mangoes are also rich in papain enzyme that helps in breaking down the protein waste in the body.

- o Watermelons can also be included in your day two diet as it is known for its diuretic properties. This will help in the quick removal of the fluids that causes toxins in your body.

- o Grapes will help in fighting with the production of mucus in your body that will clog up the tissues in the body. It will also help in cleansing the liver and the kidneys. It is one that will provide you instant energy.

Day 3

Day 3 has all the menus that you have taken or day 2 and the only change in day 3 is that you can also include raw vegetable salad for lunch and dinner. Make sure that you do not cook the vegetables and that you only take it in its raw and uncooked state. You can choose a combination of the vegetables that you like to prepare your veggie salad. But, it would be better off for you to include the following detoxification ingredients in your veggie salad to aid in digestion and also to help in detoxification of your body so that you earn a healthy body.

- o Add dandelion leaves in your veggie salad as it is loaded with diuretic properties that will help in reducing fluid retention in your body. It is also an excellent tonic for the kidneys and liver.

- o Adding fennel seeds or a pinch of freshly ground fennel powder in your salad will help in improving digestion as well as preventing flatulence.

- o Parsley is an excellent diuretic ingredient that is loaded with vitamins and minerals.

It will also help in ensuring the proper functioning of the liver.

Day 4

Day 4 is one day that you would enjoy as you get a chance to eat a meal that consists of boiled vegetables and cooked brown rice. The other meal of the day should of course be the raw vegetable salad that you had on day three. Make sure that you do not stop with the regular consumption of plain water. You can substitute one or two glasses of water with a cup or two of herbal hot green tea. Brown rice is rich in fiber and is easily digestible. It will help in soaking up the toxins in the gut. You can also stir fry your vegetables with spices and herbs to enhance its taste. Make sure that you do not add salt to your boiled or stir fried vegetables.

- o Adding leeks, onions and garlic to your vegetable salad will not just add flavor to your salad, but will also help in the elimination of the toxic metals in your body.

- o Adding artichokes in your salad will help you to stimulate the production of bile in the liver and will also help in speedy digestion.

Day 5

You can add beans and lentils in a cooked state in your day five diet. You should not eat the beans and the lentils along with any form of rice as beans are rich sources of proteins and rice is loaded with carbohydrates. Mixing proteins and starchy carbohydrate together might slow up the digestion process.

- o Make sure that you leave at least four hours of time gap between the consumption of these two foods.

- o You can also eat a handful of unsalted nuts and seeds as a midday meal. This will help to make you feel fuller for a long time. It will also help in speeding up digestion.

Day 6

You can add natural, fat free yoghurt to your detox diet on day six. This yoghurt is easily digestible and you can have it with your fresh fruit salad or oats porridge or oats with sweetened honey and nuts. You can also have the regular brown rice with tossed vegetable salad or stir fried vegetables for lunch or for dinner. Never forget to drink plenty of water and also to start your day with lemon juice or hot lemon green tea before breakfast. You can also think of going for brown noodles as your lunch or dinner along with your favorite veggie salad. As you are taking fruits and natural yoghurt, you are sure to feel fuller and might not need to eat any mid day snack.

Day 7

Day seven is the last day of your week long detox diet program. It is also going to be one of the best diet days of your seven day detox diet plan as you get a chance to add fish to one of your meals on day 7. You can eat any fresh fish that you like and it is recommended that you go for salmons or tuna or sardines as it will also help your skin from benefitting from the essential fatty acids found in these fishes. You can eat boiled or baked one serving of tuna or salmon fish along with brown rice. It would be better off for you to have this meal at lunch rather than dinner.

Some of the tips that you need to follow during your seven day detox diet program:

- o Make sure that you carry out body brushing on all the seven days of the detox program when you are having your bath. Use a loofah or a fiber body brush to brush your skin before heading or a shower on all the days.

- o Make sure that you chew the food that you eat at least 10 to 12 times before swallowing the food. This will help in easy digestion of the food and will also ensure that you do not overeat.

o It would also be better if you could detoxify your mind along with your body. You need to do at least 15 minutes of meditation every day in the morning to enjoy a healthy body and mind.